CW00518505

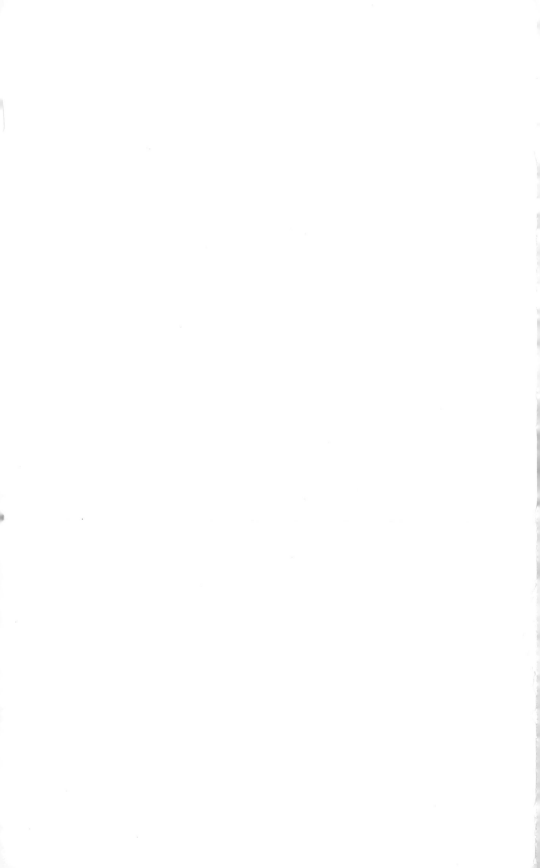

Lean and Green

Air Fryer Cookbook

2021

Super Tasty, Wholesome and Easy Air Fryer
Seafood Recipes to Losing Weight and Staying
Healthy Without Sacrificing The Taste of Meals

Aline Chang

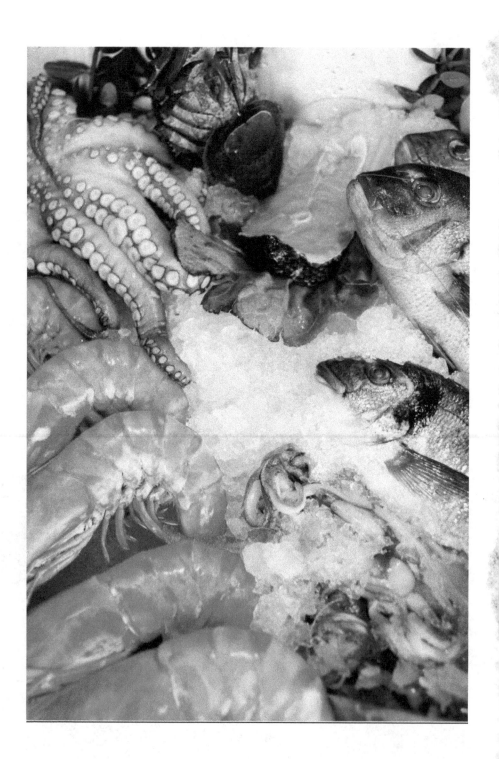

© Copyright 2021 – Aline Chang - All rights reserved.

The content contained within this book may not be reproduced, duplicated or transmitted without direct written permission from the author or the publisher. Under no circumstances will any blame or legal responsibility be held against the publisher, or author, for any damages, reparation, or monetary loss due to the information contained within this book. Either directly or indirectly.

Legal Notice

This book is copyright protected. This book is only for personal use. You cannot amend, distribute, sell, use, quote or paraphrase any part, or the content within this book, without the consent of the author or publisher.

Disclaimer Notice

Please note the information contained within this document is for educational and entertainment purposes only. All effort has been executed to present accurate, up to date, and reliable, complete information. No warranties of any kind are declared or implied. Readers acknowledge that the author is not engaging in the rendering of legal, financial, medical or professional advice. The content within this book has been derived from various sources. Please consult a licensed professional before attempting any techniques outlined in this book. By reading this document, the reader agrees that under no circumstances is the author responsible for any losses, direct or indirect, which are incurred as a result of the use of information contained within this document, including, but not limited to, — errors, omissions, or inaccuracies.

Contents

AIR FRYER SECTION

Introduction

Why Air Fryer?

If you are new to the idea of Air Frying and still struggling with the use of an Air Fryer, then continue reading, as the text of this cookbook will provide you all the Air fryer recipes. An Air Fryer can be that kitchen companion that you can use to cook a wide variety of recipes. The appliance makes frying possible without the use of excessive oil. The food placed inside the cooking chamber of an Air Fryer is exposed to hot air, which fries the food from the outside and cooks well it on the inside. This heating system is controlled with a thermostat and a control panel installed on an Air Fryer.

The recipe section of this cookbook brings you all the delicious recipes that can make your routine menu healthy and nourishing. There is no better way than to start a day with crispy bacon served with egg cups or frittata. And when you have an Air Fryer, you can cook them all in a single vessel in just a few minutes. Then you can always try making healthy snacks at home. Making crispy burgers is not a big deal when you have an Air Fryer at home. Why waste your money on the expensive fast food from outside when you can make much healthier and equally delicious meals at home.

Regular frying is all about soaking food in hot oil and leave it there until it completely cooked, browned and crispy. In this process, you need to go extra miles to get rid of all the excess oil, and still, some oil is always left in the food after frying. Due to this reason, the food cooked through regular frying usually has higher fat content, which is not always healthy, especially for those who are suffering from high cholesterol or cardiac problems. Besides, it is not easy to deal with oil frying. Hot oil can be dangerous, and it does not leave the environment clean.

Air Frying, on the other hand, does not use oil as the medium of cooking. The food is not completely dipped or soaked in the oil; rather, it is kept in a sealed chamber where hot air is passed with pressure. The high temperature and high pressure of the air create a cumulative effect that fries the food from the outside, leaving it crispy and crunchy, whereas the overall temperature within the vessel cooks the food from the inside.

Please Note: *All the recipes have been written with the most famous model of air fryer oven in mind, the Breville Oven. If you ever have another air fryer, don't worry. You can still follow the recipe to the letter, adapting the part of the Breville Air Fryer to your Air fryer Machine.*

Air Fryer Recipes

Seafood Recipes

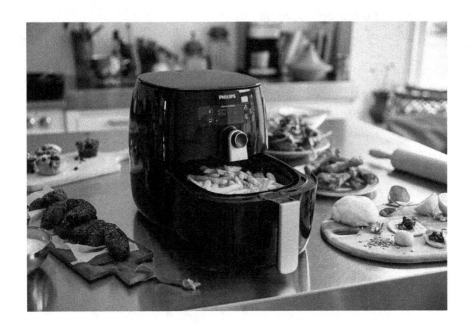

Trout Frittata

Servings: 4
Preparation Time: 15 minutes
Cooking Time: 25 minutes

Ingredients:

- 1 tablespoon olive oil
- 1 onion, sliced
- 6 eggs
- ½ tablespoon horseradish sauce
- 2 tablespoons crème fraiche
- 2 hot-smoked trout fillets, chopped
- ¼ cup fresh dill, chopped

Instructions:

1. In a skillet, heat the oil over medium heat and cook the onion for about 4-5 minutes.
2. Remove from the heat and set aside.
3. Meanwhile, in a bowl, add the eggs, horseradish sauce, and crème fraiche and mix well.
4. In the bottom of a baking dish, place the cooked onion and top with the egg mixture, followed by trout.
5. Select "Air Fry" of Breville Smart Air Fryer Oven and adjust the temperature to 320 degrees F.
6. Set the timer for 20 minutes and press "Start/Stop" to begin preheating.
7. When the unit beeps to show that it is preheated, arrange the baking dish over the wire rack.

8. When the cooking time is completed, remove the baking dish from oven and place onto a wire rack to cool for about 5 minutes before serving.
9. Cut into equal-sized wedges and serve with the garnishing of dill.

Nutritional Information per Serving:

Calories: 288
Fat: 19.2g
Carbohydrates: 5.1g
Fiber: 1g
Sugar: 1.8g
Protein: 22.4g
Sodium: 144mg

Simple Trout

Servings: 2
Preparation Time: 10 minutes
Cooking Time: 10 minutes

Ingredients:

- 2 (6-ounce) trout fillets
- Salt and ground black pepper, as required
- 1 tablespoon olive oil
- 3 cups fresh baby spinach

Instructions:

1. Season each trout fillet with salt and black pepper and then coat with the oil.
2. Arrange the trout fillets onto the greased enamel roasting pan in a single layer.
3. Select "Air Fry" of Breville Smart Air Fryer Oven and adjust the temperature to 360 degrees F.
4. Set the timer for 10 minutes and press "Start/Stop" to begin preheating.
5. When the unit beeps to show that it is preheated, insert the roasting pan in the oven.
6. Flip the fillets once halfway through.
7. When the cooking time is completed, remove the roasting pan from the oven and transfer the trout fillets onto serving plates.
8. Serve hot alongside the spinach.

Nutritional Information per Serving:

Calories: 276
Fat: 12.9g
Carbohydrates: 1.6g
Fiber: 1g
Sugar: 0.2g
Protein: 36.7g
Sodium: 164mg

Salmon Quiche

Servings: 3
Preparation Time: 15 minutes
Cooking Time: 20 minutes

Ingredients:

- 5½ ounces salmon fillet, chopped
- Salt and ground black pepper, as required
- ½ tablespoon fresh lemon juice
- 1 egg yolk
- 3½ tablespoons chilled coconut oil
- 2/3 cup almond flour
- 1 tablespoon cold water
- 2 eggs
- 3 tablespoons whipping cream
- 1 scallion, chopped

Instructions:

1. In a bowl, add the salmon, salt, black pepper and lemon juice and mix well.
2. In another bowl, add the egg yolk, coconut oil, flour and water and mix until a dough forms.
3. Place the dough onto a floured smooth surface and roll into about 7-inch round.
4. Place the dough in a quiche pan and press firmly in the bottom and along the edges.
5. Trim the excess edges.

6. In a small bowl, add the eggs, cream, salt and black pepper and beat until well combined.
7. Place the cream mixture over the crust evenly and top with the salmon mixture, followed by the scallion.
8. Select "Air Fry" of Breville Smart Air Fryer Oven and adjust the temperature to 355 degrees F.
9. Set the timer for 20 minutes and press "Start/Stop" to begin preheating.
10. When the unit beeps to show that it is preheated, arrange the quiche pan over the wire rack.
11. When the cooking time is completed, remove the quiche pan from the oven and set aside for about 5 minutes before serving.
12. Cut the quiche into equal-sized wedges and serve.

Nutritional Information per Serving:

Calories: 471
Fat: 41.5g
Carbohydrates: 5.7g
Fiber: 2.8g
Sugar: 1.3g
Protein: 15.1g
Sodium: 124mg

Salmon & Veggie Stew

Servings: 4
Preparation Time: 15 minutes
Cooking Time: 6 hours

Ingredients:

- 1-pound salmon fillet, cubed
- 1 tablespoon coconut oil
- 1 medium yellow onion, chopped
- 1 garlic clove, minced
- 1 zucchini, sliced
- 1 green bell pepper, seeded and cubed
- ½ cup tomatoes, chopped
- ½ cup fish broth
- ¼ teaspoon dried oregano
- ¼ teaspoon dried basil
- Salt and ground black pepper, as required

Instructions:

1. In an oven-safe pan that will fit in the Breville Smart Air Fryer Oven, place all ingredients and stir to combine.
2. Cover the pan with a lid.
3. Arrange the pan over the wire rack.
4. Select "Slow Cooker" of Breville Smart Air Fryer Oven and set on "Low".
5. Set the timer for 5-6 hours and press "Start/Stop" to begin cooking.

6. When the cooking time is completed, remove the pan from the oven and serve hot.

Nutritional Information per Serving:

Calories: 218
Fat: 10.9g
Carbohydrates: 7.7g
Fiber: 5.4g
Sugar: 4.1g
Protein: 24.1g
Sodium: 142mg

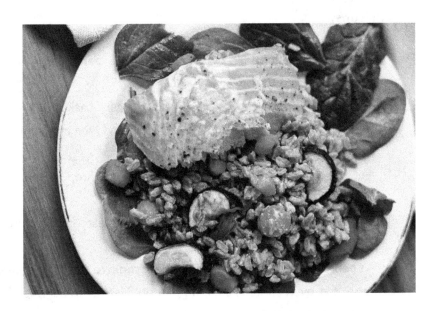

Simple Salmon

Servings: 2
Preparation Time: 10 minutes
Cooking Time: 10 minutes

Ingredients:

- 2 (6-ounce) salmon fillets
- Salt and ground black pepper, as required
- 1 tablespoon olive oil
- 3 cups fresh baby spinach

Instructions:

1. Season each salmon fillet with salt and black pepper and then coat with the oil.
2. Arrange the salmon fillets into the greased air fry basket.
3. Select "Air Fry" of Breville Smart Air Fryer Oven and adjust the temperature to 360 degrees F.
4. Set the timer for 10 minutes and press "Start/Stop" to begin preheating.
5. When the unit beeps to show that it is preheated, insert the air fry basket in the oven.
6. When the cooking time is completed, remove the air fry basket from the oven and transfer the salmon fillets onto serving plates.
7. Serve hot alongside the spinach.

Nutritional Information per Serving:

Calories: 218
Fat: 10.9g
Carbohydrates: 7.7g
Fiber: 5.4g
Sugar: 4.1g
Protein: 24.1g
Sodium: 142mg

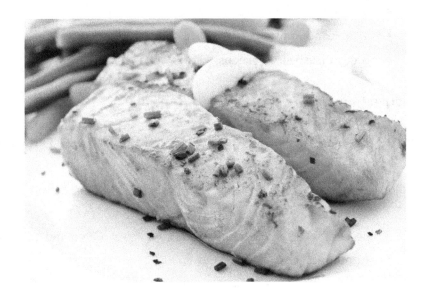

Cajun Salmon

Servings: 2
Preparation Time: 10 minutes
Cooking Time: 7 minutes

Ingredients:

- 2 (7-ounce) (¾-inch thick) salmon fillets
- 1 tablespoon Cajun seasoning
- ½ teaspoon Erythritol
- 1 tablespoon fresh lemon juice
- 3 cups fresh salad greens

Instructions:

1. Sprinkle the salmon fillets with Cajun seasoning and Erythritol evenly.
2. Arrange the salmon fillets into the greased air fry basket, skin-side up.
3. Select "Air Fry" of Breville Smart Air Fryer Oven and adjust the temperature to 356 degrees F.
4. Set the timer for 7 minutes and press "Start/Stop" to begin preheating.
5. When the unit beeps to show that it is preheated, insert the air fry basket in the oven.
6. When the cooking time is completed, remove the air fry basket from the oven and transfer the salmon fillets onto serving plates.
7. Drizzle with the lemon juice and serve hot alongside the salad greens.

Nutritional Information per Serving:

Calories: 276
Fat: 12.5g
Carbohydrates: 2.6g
Fiber: 0.6g
Sugar: 1g
Protein: 39g
Sodium: 169mg

Spicy Salmon

Servings: 2
Preparation Time: 10 minutes
Cooking Time: 11 minutes

Ingredients:

- 1 teaspoon smoked paprika
- 1 teaspoon cayenne pepper
- 1 teaspoon onion powder
- 1 teaspoon garlic powder
- Salt and ground black pepper, as required
- 2 (6-ounce) (1½-inch thick) salmon fillets
- 2 teaspoons olive oil
- 3 cups fresh spinach

Instructions:

1. In a bowl, add the spices, salt and black pepper and mix well.
2. Drizzle the salmon fillets with oil and then rub with the spice mixture.
3. Arrange the salmon fillets into the greased air fry basket, skin-side up.
4. Select "Air Fry" of Breville Smart Air Fryer Oven and adjust the temperature to 390 degrees F.
5. Set the timer for 11 minutes and press "Start/Stop" to begin preheating.
6. When the unit beeps to show that it is preheated, insert the air fry basket in the oven.

7. When the cooking time is completed, remove the air fry basket from the oven and transfer the salmon fillets onto serving plates.

8. Serve hot alongside the spinach.

Nutritional Information per Serving:

Calories: 290
Fat: 15.7g
Carbohydrates: 4.7g
Fiber: 1.8g
Sugar: 1.2g
Protein: 34.9g
Sodium: 189mg

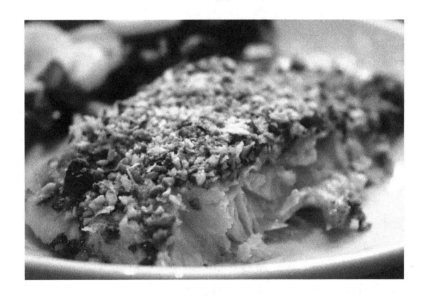

Lemony Salmon

Servings: 2
Preparation Time: 10 minutes
Cooking Time: 10 minutes

Ingredients:

- 1 tablespoon fresh lemon juice
- ½ tablespoons olive oil
- Salt and ground black pepper, as required
- 1 garlic clove, minced
- ½ teaspoon fresh thyme leaves, chopped
- 2 (7-ounce) salmon fillets
- 3 cups fresh salad greens

Instructions:

1. In a bowl, add all the ingredients except the salmon and greens and mix well.
2. Add the salmon fillets and coat with the mixture generously.
3. Coat the fillets with flour mixture, then dip into egg mixture and finally coat with the cornflake mixture.
4. Arrange the salmon fillets onto a lightly greased wire rack, skin-side down.
5. Select "Air Fry" of Breville Smart Air Fryer Oven and adjust the temperature to 400 degrees F.
6. Set the timer for 10 minutes and press "Start/Stop" to begin preheating.
7. When the unit beeps to show that it is preheated, insert the wire rack in the oven.

8. Flip the salmon fillets once halfway through.
9. When the cooking time is completed, remove the salmon fillets from the oven and transfer onto serving plates.
10. Serve hot alongside the greens.

Nutritional Information per Serving:

Calories: 309
Fat: 16g
Carbohydrates: 3.3g
Fiber: 0.7g
Sugar: 1g
Protein: 39.1g
Sodium: 171mg

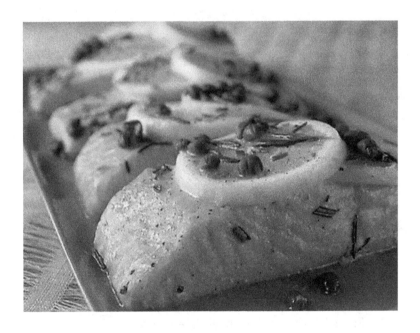

Pesto Salmon

Servings: 4
Preparation Time: 15 minutes
Cooking Time: 15 minutes

Ingredients:

For Salmon:

- 1¼ pounds salmon fillet, cut into 4 fillets
- 2 tablespoons fresh lemon juice
- 2 tablespoons pesto, thawed

For Serving:

- 1 cucumber, chopped
- 1 large tomato, chopped

Instructions:

1. Arrange the salmon fillets onto a foil-lined baking dish, skin-side down.
2. Drizzle the salmon fillets with lemon juice.
3. Set aside for about 15 minutes.
4. Spread pesto over each salmon fillet evenly.
5. Arrange the salmon fillets into the greased baking dish.
6. Select "Broil" of Breville Smart Air Fryer Oven and then set the timer for 15 minutes.
7. Press "Start/Stop" to begin preheating.
8. When the unit beeps to show that it is preheated, arrange the baking dish over the wire rack.

9. When the cooking time is completed, remove the baking dish from oven and transfer the salmon fillets onto serving plates.

10. Serve hot alongside cucumber and tomato.

Nutritional Information per Serving:

Calories: 243
Fat: 12.2g
Carbohydrates: 5.2g
Fiber: 1.1g
Sugar: 3.1g
Protein: 29.2g
Sodium: 115mg

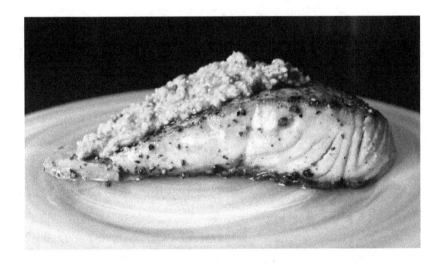

Honey Glazed Salmon

Servings: 2
Preparation Time: 10 minutes
Cooking Time: 8 minutes

Ingredients:

- 2 (6-ounce) salmon fillets
- Salt, as required
- 2 tablespoons honey
- 3 cups fresh baby kale

Instructions:

1. Sprinkle the salmon fillets with salt and then coat with honey.
2. Arrange the salmon fillets into the greased air fry basket, skin-side up.
3. Select "Air Fry" of Breville Smart Air Fryer Oven and adjust the temperature to 355 degrees F.
4. Set the timer for 8 minutes and press "Start/Stop" to begin preheating.
5. When the unit beeps to show that it is preheated, insert the air fry basket in the oven.
6. When the cooking time is completed, remove the air fry basket from the oven and transfer the salmon fillets onto serving plates.
7. Serve hot alongside the kale.

Nutritional Information per Serving:

Calories: 323

Fat: 10.9g

Carbohydrates: 19.1g

Fiber: 1.5g

Sugar: 16g

Protein: 35.3g

Sodium: 180mg

Sweet & Sour Salmon

Servings: 2
Preparation Time: 10 minutes
Cooking Time: 13 minutes

Ingredients:

- 3 tablespoons low-sodium soy sauce
- 2 tablespoons maple syrup
- 2 teaspoons fresh lemon juice
- 2 teaspoons water
- 2 (4-ounce) salmon fillets
- 3 cups fresh arugula

Instructions:

1. In a small bowl, place all the ingredients except the salmon and arugula and mix well.
2. In a small bowl, reserve about half of the sauce mixture.
3. Add the salmon in the remaining mixture and coat well.
4. Refrigerate, covered to marinate for about 2 hours.
5. Arrange the salmon fillets into the greased air fry basket.
6. Select "Air Fry" of Breville Smart Air Fryer Oven and adjust the temperature to 355 degrees F.
7. Set the timer for 13 minutes and press "Start/Stop" to begin preheating.
8. When the unit beeps to show that it is preheated, insert the air fry basket in the oven.
9. After 8 minutes, flip the salmon fillets and coat with reserved marinade.

10. When the cooking time is completed, remove the air fry basket from the oven and serve hot alongside the arugula.

Nutritional Information per Serving:

Calories: 218
Fat: 7.3g
Carbohydrates: 15g
Fiber: 0.5g
Sugar: 14.1g
Protein: 24.3g
Sodium: 1089mg

Salmon Parcel

Servings: 2
Preparation Time: 15 minutes
Cooking Time: 23 minutes

Ingredients:

- 2 (4-ounce) salmon fillets
- 8 asparagus stalks
- ¼ cup white sauce
- 1 tablespoon oil
- ¼ cup low-sodium chicken broth
- Salt and ground black pepper, as required

Instructions:

1. In a bowl, mix together all the ingredients.
2. Divide the salmon mixture over 2 pieces of foil evenly.
3. Seal the foil around the salmon mixture to form the packet.
4. Arrange the salmon parcels in air fry basket.
5. Select "Air Fry" of Breville Smart Air Fryer Oven and adjust the temperature to 355 degrees F.
6. Set the timer for 13 minutes and press "Start/Stop" to begin preheating.
7. When the unit beeps to show that it is preheated, insert the air fry basket in the oven.
8. When the cooking time is completed, remove the air fry basket from the oven and transfer the parcels onto serving plates.
9. Carefully open the parcels and serve hot.

Nutritional Information per Serving:

Calories: 265
Fat: 17.2g
Carbohydrates: 4.3g
Fiber: 0.8g
Sugar: 2g
Protein: 24.2g
Sodium: 248mg

Salmon in Dill Sauce

Servings: 6
Preparation Time: 10 minutes
Cooking Time: 2 hours

Ingredients:

- 2 cups water
- 1 cup low-sodium chicken broth
- 2 tablespoons fresh lemon juice
- ¼ cup fresh dill, chopped
- ½ teaspoon lemon zest, grated
- 6 (4-ounce) salmon fillets
- 1 teaspoon cayenne pepper
- Salt and ground black pepper, as required
- 8 cups fresh baby kale

Instructions:

1. In an oven-safe pan that will fit in the Breville Smart Air Fryer Oven, mix together the water, broth, lemon juice, dill and lemon zest.
2. Arrange the salmon fillets on top, skin side down and sprinkle with cayenne pepper, salt black pepper.
3. Cover the pan with a lid.
4. Arrange the pan over the wire rack.
5. Select "Slow Cooker" of Breville Smart Air Fryer Oven and set on "Low".
6. Set the timer for 2 hours and press "Start/Stop" to begin cooking.

7. When the cooking time is completed, remove the pan from the oven.
8. Remove the lid and serve hot alongside the kale.

Nutritional Information per Serving:

Calories: 204
Fat: 7.2g
Carbohydrates: 10g
Fiber: 1.7g
Sugar: 0.2g
Protein: 25.2g
Sodium: 135mg

Salmon with Broccoli

Servings: 2
Preparation Time: 15 minutes
Cooking Time: 12 minutes

Ingredients:

- 1 ½ cups small broccoli florets
- 2 tablespoons olive oil, divided
- Salt and ground black pepper, as required
- 1 (½-inch) piece fresh ginger, grated
- 1 tablespoon low-sodium soy sauce
- 1 teaspoon balsamic vinegar
- 1 teaspoon Erythritol
- ¼ teaspoon arrowroot starch
- 2 (6-ounce) skin-on salmon fillets
- 1 scallion, thinly sliced

Instructions:

1. In a bowl, mix together the broccoli, 1 tablespoon of oil, salt, and black pepper.
2. In another bowl, mix well the ginger, soy sauce, vinegar, Erythritol, and cornstarch.
3. Coat the salmon fillets with the remaining oil and then with the ginger mixture.
4. Arrange the broccoli florets into the greased air fry basket and top with the salmon fillets.
5. Select "Air Fry" of Breville Smart Air Fryer Oven and adjust the temperature to 375 degrees F.

6. Set the timer for 12 minutes and press "Start/Stop" to begin preheating.
7. When the unit beeps to show that it is preheated, insert the air fry basket in the oven.
8. When the cooking time is completed, remove the air fry basket from the oven and transfer the salmon fillets and broccoli onto serving plates.
9. Serve hot.

Nutritional Information per Serving:

Calories: 375
Fat: 24.7g
Carbohydrates: 5.9g
Fiber: 2g
Sugar: 1.8g
Protein: 35.6g
Sodium: 539mg

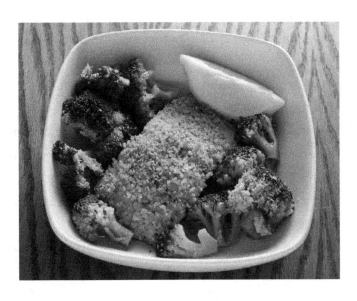

Salmon with Asparagus

Servings: 2
Preparation Time: 15 minutes
Cooking Time: 11 minutes

Ingredients:

- 2 (6-ounces) boneless salmon fillets
- 1½ tablespoons fresh lemon juice
- 1 tablespoon olive oil
- 2 tablespoons fresh parsley, roughly chopped
- 2 tablespoons fresh dill, roughly chopped
- 1 bunch asparagus
- Salt and ground black pepper, as required

Instructions:

1. In a small bowl, mix well the lemon juice, oil, herbs, salt, and black pepper.
2. In another large bowl, mix together the salmon and ¾ of oil mixture.
3. In a second large bowl, add the asparagus and remaining oil mixture and mix well.
4. Arrange the asparagus into the greased air fry basket.
5. Select "Air Fry" of Breville Smart Air Fryer Oven and adjust the temperature to 400 degrees F.
6. Set the timer for 11 minutes and press "Start/Stop" to begin preheating.
7. When the unit beeps to show that it is preheated, insert the air fry basket in the oven.

8. After 3 minutes of cooking, place the salmon fillets on top of the asparagus
9. When the cooking time is completed, remove the air fry basket from the oven and serve hot.

Nutritional Information per Serving:

Calories: 331
Fat: 18g
Carbohydrates: 8.8g
Fiber: 4.2g
Sugar: 3.5g
Protein: 37.6g
Sodium: 16mg

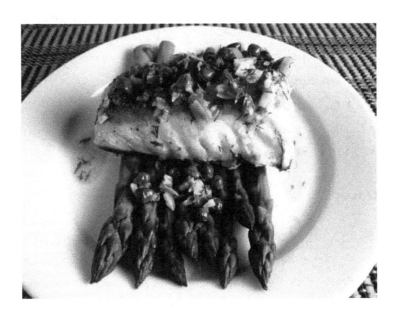

Salmon with Green Beans

Servings: 4
Preparation Time: 15 minutes
Cooking Time: 12 minutes

Ingredients:

For Green Beans

- 5 cups green beans
- 1 tablespoon avocado oil
- Salt, as required

For Salmon

- 2 garlic cloves, minced
- 2 tablespoons fresh dill, chopped
- 2 tablespoons fresh lemon juice
- 1 tablespoon olive oil
- Salt, as required
- 4 (6-ounces) salmon fillets

Instructions:

1. In a large bowl, mix together the green beans, oil, and salt.
2. Arrange the green beans into the greased air fry basket.
3. Select "Air Fry" of Breville Smart Air Fryer Oven and adjust the temperature to 375 degrees F.
4. Set the timer for 12 minutes and press "Start/Stop" to begin preheating.

5. When the unit beeps to show that it is preheated, insert the air fry basket in the oven.

6. After 6 minutes of cooking, flip the green beans and top with salmon fillets.

7. Place the garlic mixture on top of each salmon fillet evenly and then, sprinkle with the salt.

8. When the cooking time is completed, remove the air fry basket from the oven and place the salmon fillets onto serving plates.

9. Serve hot alongside the green beans.

Nutritional Information per Serving:

Calories: 310
Fat: 14.8g
Carbohydrates: 11.1g
Fiber: 5.1g
Sugar: 2.1g
Protein: 36g
Sodium: 128mg

Simple Cod

Servings: 4
Preparation Time: 10 minutes
Cooking Time: 12 minutes

Ingredients:

- 4 (6-ounce) cod fillets
- Salt and ground black pepper, as required
- 6 cups fresh arugula

Instructions:

1. Season the cod fillets with salt and black pepper evenly.
2. Arrange the cod fillets over the greased wire rack.
3. Select "Broil" of Breville Smart Air Fryer Oven and set the timer for 15 minutes.
4. Press "Start/Stop" to begin preheating.
5. When the unit beeps to show that it is preheated, insert the wire rack in the oven.
6. When the cooking time is completed, remove the wire rack from the oven and transfer the cod fillets onto serving plates.
7. Serve hot alongside the arugula.

Nutritional Information per Serving:

Calories: 144
Fat: 1.7g
Carbohydrates: 1.1g
Fiber: 0.5g
Sugar: 0.6g
Protein: 31.1g
Sodium: 153mg

Cod with Asparagus

Servings: 1
Preparation Time: 10 minutes
Cooking Time: 15 minutes

Ingredients:

- 1 (6-ounce) cod fillet
- Salt and ground black pepper, as required
- 6 asparagus spears, trimmed
- 1 teaspoon olive oil
- 1 tablespoon fresh lemon juice

Instructions:

1. Season the cod fillet with salt and black pepper.
2. In a small bowl, add the asparagus, salt, black pepper and oil and toss to coat well.
3. Arrange the cod fillet into a greased baking dish on 1 side.
4. Arrange the asparagus spears alongside the cod fillet.
5. Select "Bake" of Breville Smart Air Fryer Oven and adjust the temperature to 450 degrees F.
6. Set the timer for 15 minutes and press "Start/Stop" to begin preheating.
7. When the unit beeps to show that it is preheated, arrange the baking dish over the wire rack.
8. When the cooking time is completed, remove the baking dish from oven and transfer the cod fillet and asparagus onto a serving plate.
9. Drizzle with lemon juice and serve immediately.

Nutritional Information per Serving:

Calories: 209
Fat: 6.5g
Carbohydrates: 5.9g
Fiber: 3.1g
Sugar: 3g
Protein: 33.7g
Sodium: 267mg

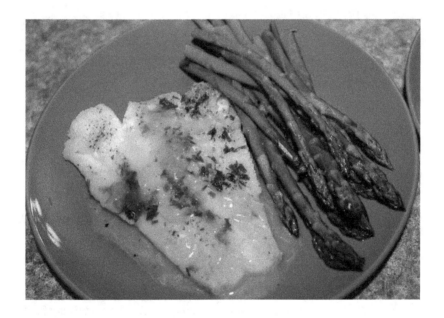

Cod & Veggie Parcel

Servings: 2
Preparation Time: 15 minutes
Cooking Time: 20 minutes

Ingredients:

- 3 tablespoons olive oil, divided
- 1 tablespoon fresh lemon juice
- ½ teaspoon dried tarragon
- Salt and ground black pepper, as required
- ½ cup red bell peppers, seeded and thinly sliced
- ½ cup carrots, peeled and julienned
- ½ cup fennel bulbs, julienned
- 2 (5-ounce) frozen cod fillets, thawed

Instructions:

1. In a large bowl, mix together 2 tablespoons of the oil, lemon juice, tarragon, salt, and black pepper.
2. Add the bell pepper, carrot, and fennel bulb and generously coat with the mixture.
3. Arrange 2 large parchment squares onto a smooth surface.
4. Coat the cod fillets with remaining oil and then sprinkle evenly with salt and black pepper.
5. Arrange 1 cod fillet onto each parchment square and top each evenly with the vegetables.
6. Top with any remaining sauce from the bowl.
7. Fold the parchment paper and crimp the sides to secure fish and vegetables.

8. Arrange the cod parcels into the air fry basket.
9. Select "Air Fry" of Breville Smart Air Fryer Oven and adjust the temperature to 350 degrees F.
10. Set the timer for 15 minutes and press "Start/Stop" to begin preheating.
11. When the unit beeps to show that it is preheated, insert the air fry basket in the oven.
12. When the cooking time is completed, remove the air fry basket from the oven and transfer the parcels onto serving plates.
13. Carefully open the parcels and serve hot.

Nutritional Information per Serving:

Calories: 324
Fat: 22.5g
Carbohydrates: 6.8g
Fiber: 1.8g
Sugar: 3g
Protein: 26.2g
Sodium: 199mg

Cod Burgers

Servings: 6
Preparation Time: 15 minutes
Cooking Time: 7 minutes

Ingredients:

- 1-pound cod fillet
- 1 teaspoon fresh lime zest, finely grated
- 1 egg
- 1 teaspoon red chili paste
- Salt, as required
- 1 tablespoon fresh lime juice
- 1/3 cup coconut, grated and divided
- 1 scallion, finely chopped
- 2 tablespoons fresh parsley, chopped
- 6 cups fresh baby greens
- 1½ cups cherry tomatoes, halved

Instructions:

1. For cod patties: in a food processor, add the cod fillet, lime zest, egg, chili paste, salt, and lime juice and pulse until smooth.
2. Transfer the cod mixture into a bowl.
3. Add 2 tablespoons of coconut, scallion, and parsley and mix until well combined.
4. Make 12 equal-sized patties from the mixture.
5. In a shallow bowl, place the remaining coconut.
6. Coat the cod patties with coconut evenly.
7. Arrange the patties into the greased air fry basket.

8. Select "Air Fry" of Breville Smart Air Fryer Oven and adjust the temperature to 375 degrees F.
9. Set the timer for 7 minutes and press "Start/Stop" to begin preheating.
10. When the unit beeps to show that it is preheated, insert the air fry basket in the oven.
11. When the cooking time is completed, remove the air fry basket from the oven and serve alongside the greens and tomatoes.

Nutritional Information per Serving:

Calories: 103
Fat: 3.1g
Carbohydrates: 3.8g
Fiber: 1.4g
Sugar: 2.2g
Protein: 15.5g
Sodium: 102mg

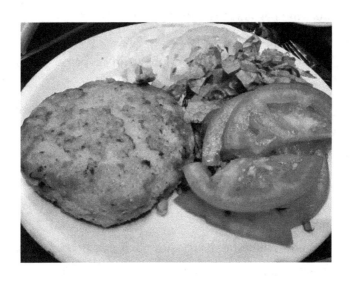

Tangy Sea Bass

Servings: 2
Preparation Time: 10 minutes
Cooking Time: 12 minutes

Ingredients:

- 2 (5-ounce) sea bass fillets
- 1 garlic clove, minced
- 1 teaspoon fresh dill, minced
- 1 tablespoon olive oil
- 1 tablespoon balsamic vinegar
- Salt and ground black pepper, as required
- 3 cups fresh baby spinach

Instructions:

1. In a large resealable bag, add all the ingredients.
2. Seal the bag and shale well to mix.
3. Refrigerate to marinate for at least 30 minutes.
4. Remove the fish fillets from bag and shake off the excess marinade.
5. Arrange the fish fillets onto the greased enamel roasting pan in a single layer.
6. Select "Bake" of Breville Smart Air Fryer Oven and adjust the temperature to 450 degrees F.
7. Set the timer for 12 minutes and press "Start/Stop" to begin preheating.
8. When the unit beeps to show that it is preheated, insert the roasting pan in the oven.

9. Flip the fish fillets once halfway through.
10. When the cooking time is completed, remove the roasting pan from the oven and transfer the fish fillets onto serving plates.
11. Serve hot alongside the spinach.

Nutritional Information per Serving:

Calories: 251
Fat: 10.8g
Carbohydrates: 2.5g
Fiber: 1.1g
Sugar: 0.2g
Protein: 35g
Sodium: 238mg

Spiced Tilapia

Servings: 2
Preparation Time: 10 minutes
Cooking Time: 12 minutes

Ingredients:

- ½ teaspoon lemon pepper seasoning
- ½ teaspoon garlic powder
- 1/2 teaspoon onion powder
- Salt and ground black pepper, as required
- 2 (6-ounce) tilapia fillets
- 1 tablespoon olive oil
- 3 cups fresh spinach

Instructions:

1. In a small bowl, mix together the spices, salt and black pepper.
2. Coat the tilapia fillets with oil and then rub with spice mixture.
3. Arrange the tilapia fillets onto a lightly greased wire rack, skin-side down.
4. Select "Air Fry" of Breville Smart Air Fryer Oven and adjust the temperature to 360 degrees F.
5. Set the timer for 12 minutes and press "Start/Stop" to begin preheating.
6. When the unit beeps to show that it is preheated, insert the wire rack in the oven.
7. Flip the tilapia fillets once hallway through.
8. When the cooking time is completed, remove the tilapia fillets from the oven and transfer onto serving plates.

9. Serve hot alongside the spinach.

Nutritional Information per Serving:

Calories: 216
Fat: 8.8g
Carbohydrates: 3g
Fiber: 1.2g
Sugar: 0.6g
Protein: 33.2g
Sodium: 174mg

Ranch Tilapia

Servings: 4
Preparation Time: 10 minutes
Cooking Time: 13 minutes

Ingredients:

- ¾ cup cornflakes, crushed
- 1 (1-ounce) packet dry ranch-style dressing mix
- 2½ tablespoons olive oil
- 2 eggs
- 4 (6-ounce) tilapia fillets
- 6 cups fresh salad greens

Instructions:

1. In a shallow bowl, beat the eggs.
2. In another bowl, add the cornflakes, ranch dressing, and oil and mix until a crumbly mixture forms.
3. Dip the fish fillets into egg and then coat with the breadcrumbs mixture.
4. Arrange the tilapia fillets into the greased air fry basket.
5. Select "Air Fry" of Breville Smart Air Fryer Oven and adjust the temperature to 356 degrees F.
6. Set the timer for 13 minutes and press "Start/Stop" to begin preheating.
7. When the unit beeps to show that it is preheated, insert the air fry basket in the oven.
8. When the cooking time is completed, remove the tilapia fillets from the oven and transfer onto serving plates.

9. Serve hot alongside the greens.

Nutritional Information per Serving:

Calories: 302
Fat: 15g
Carbohydrates: 7.4g
Fiber: 0.7g
Sugar: 1.6g
Protein: 35.2g
Sodium: 165mg

Gingered Halibut

Servings: 4
Preparation Time: 15 minutes
Cooking Time: 30 minutes

Ingredients:

- 1-pound halibut fillets
- 1 tablespoon ginger paste
- 1 tablespoon garlic paste
- Salt and ground black pepper, as required
- 6 cups fresh spinach

Instructions:

1. Coat the halibut fillets with ginger-garlic paste and then season with salt and black pepper.
2. Arrange the halibut fillets into the greased air fry basket.
3. Select "Bake" of Breville Smart Air Fryer Oven and adjust the temperature to 380 degrees F.
4. Set the timer for 30 minutes and press "Start/Stop" to begin preheating.
5. When the unit beeps to show that it is preheated, insert the air fry basket in the oven.
6. When the cooking time is completed, remove the remove the halibut fillets from the oven and transfer onto serving plates.
7. Serve hot alongside the spinach.

Nutritional Information per Serving:

Calories: 144
Fat: 2.9g
Carbohydrates: 3.3g
Fiber: 1.2g
Sugar: 0.3g
Protein: 25.4g
Sodium: 135mg

Tangy Halibut

Servings: 2
Preparation Time: 15 minutes
Cooking Time: 12 minutes

Ingredients:

- 2 (5-ounce) halibut fillets
- 1 garlic clove, minced
- 1 teaspoon fresh rosemary, minced
- 1 tablespoon olive oil
- 1 tablespoon balsamic vinegar
- 1/8 teaspoon hot sauce
- 3 cups fresh baby greens

Instructions:

1. In a large resealable bag, add all the ingredients except for greens.
2. Seal the bag and shale well to mix.
3. Refrigerate to marinate for at least 30 minutes.
4. Line a baking pan with a piece of foil.
5. Remove the fish fillets from bag and shake off the excess marinade.
6. Arrange the fish fillets into the prepared baking pan.
7. Arrange the pan over the wire rack.
8. Select "Bake" of Breville Smart Air Fryer Oven and adjust the temperature to 450 degrees F.
9. Set the timer for 12 minutes and press "Start/Stop" to begin preheating.

10. When the unit beeps to show that it is preheated, insert the wire rack in the oven.
11. When the cooking time is completed, remove the pan from the oven and serve alongside the greens.

Nutritional Information per Serving:

Calories: 228
Fat: 10.4g
Carbohydrates: 2g
Fiber: 0.8g
Sugar: 0.6g
Protein: 30.5g
Sodium: 89mg

Sweet & Sour Halibut

Servings: 4
Preparation Time: 10 minutes
Cooking Time: 12 minutes

Ingredients:

- 4 (5-ounce) halibut fillets
- 2 garlic clove, minced
- 1 tablespoon fresh dill, minced
- 2 tablespoons olive oil
- 2 tablespoons fresh lime juice
- ½ teaspoon honey
- ¼ teaspoon Sriracha
- 6 cups fresh baby kale

Instructions:

1. In a large resealable bag, place all the ingredients except for baby kale and seal the bag.
2. Shake the bag well to mix.
3. Place the bag in the refrigerator to marinate for at least 30 minutes.
4. Remove the fish fillets from the bag and shake off the excess marinade.
5. Arrange the halibut fillets onto the greased enamel roasting pan.
6. Select "Bake" of Breville Smart Air Fryer Oven and adjust the temperature to 400 degrees F.
7. Set the timer for 12 minutes and press "Start/Stop" to begin preheating.

8. When the unit beeps to show that it is preheated, arrange the roasting pan over the wire rack.
9. When the cooking time is completed, remove the roasting pan from the oven and transfer the fish fillets onto serving plates.
10. Serve hot alongside the baby kale.

Nutritional Information per Serving:

Calories: 259
Fat: 10.8g
Carbohydrates: 8.5g
Fiber: 1.6g
Sugar: 0.7g
Protein: 32.4g
Sodium: 105mg

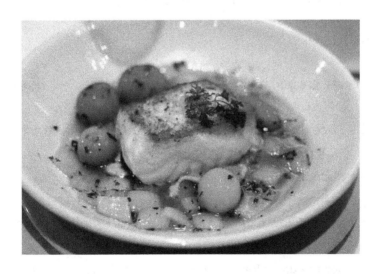

Halibut with Bell Peppers

Servings: 4
Preparation Time: 15 minutes
Cooking Time: 4 minutes

Ingredients:

- 1 green bell pepper, seeded and chopped
- 2 tomatoes, chopped
- 1 small onion, diced
- 2 garlic cloves, minced
- 1-pound halibut fillets
- 1 teaspoon dried rosemary
- Salt and ground black pepper, as required
- 1/3 cup low-sodium chicken broth

Instructions:

1. In a greased baking dish, place the tomatoes, bell pepper, onion and garlic and stir to combine.
2. Place the fish fillets on top of the tomato mixture and sprinkle with the herbs, salt and black pepper.
3. Place the broth on top evenly.
4. Arrange the baking dish over the wire rack.
5. Select "Slow Cooker" of Breville Smart Air Fryer Oven and set on "High".
6. Set the timer for 3-4 hours and press "Start/Stop" to begin cooking.
7. When the cooking time is completed, remove the pan from the oven and serve hot.

Nutritional Information per Serving:

Calories: 158
Fat: 2.9g
Carbohydrates: 7g
Fiber: 1.7g
Sugar: 3.9g
Protein: 25.2g
Sodium: 109mg

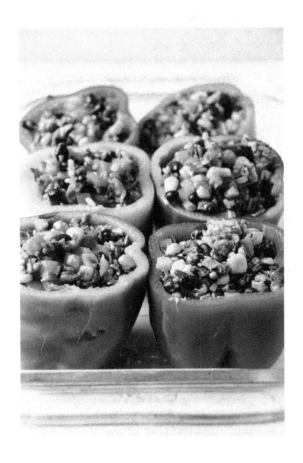

Simple Haddock

Servings: 2
Preparation Time: 10 minutes
Cooking Time: 8 minutes

Ingredients:

- 2 (6-ounces) haddock fillets
- 1 tablespoon olive oil
- Salt and ground black pepper, as required
- 3 cups fresh baby spinach

Instructions:

1. Coat the fish fillets with oil and then sprinkle with salt and black pepper.
2. Arrange fish fillets into the greased air fry basket in a single layer.
3. Select "Air Fry" of Breville Smart Air Fryer Oven and adjust the temperature to 355 degrees F.
4. Set the timer for 8 minutes and press "Start/Stop" to begin preheating.
5. When the unit beeps to show that it is preheated, insert the air fry basket in the oven.
6. When the cooking time is completed, remove the fish fillets from the oven and transfer onto serving plates.
7. Serve hot alongside the spinach.

Nutritional Information per Serving:

Calories: 261
Fat: 8.8g
Carbohydrates: 1.6g
Fiber: 1g
Sugar: 0.2g
Protein: 42.5g
Sodium: 261mg

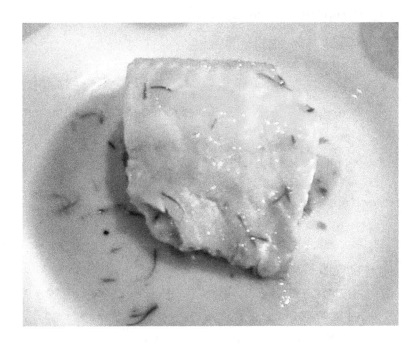

Glazed Haddock

Servings: 4
Preparation Time: 15 minutes
Cooking Time: 11 minutes

Ingredients:

- 1 garlic clove, minced
- ¼ teaspoon fresh ginger, grated finely
- ½ cup low-sodium soy sauce
- ¼ cup fresh lime juice
- ½ cup chicken broth
- ¼ cup Erythritol
- ¼ teaspoon red pepper flakes, crushed
- 1-pound haddock steaks
- 6 cups fresh baby spinach

Instructions:

1. In a pan, place all ingredients except for haddock steaks and spinach and cook for about 3-4 minutes, stirring continuously.
2. Remove from the heat and transfer the mixture into a bowl. Set aside to cool.
3. In a bowl, reserve half of the marinade.
4. In a resealable bag, add the remaining marinade and haddock steak.
5. Seal the bag and shake to coat well.
6. Refrigerate for about 30 minutes.
7. Arrange the haddock steaks into the greased air fry basket.

8. Select "Air Fry" of Breville Smart Air Fryer Oven and adjust the temperature to 390 degrees F.
9. Set the timer for 11 minutes and press "Start/Stop" to begin preheating.
10. When the unit beeps to show that it is preheated, insert the air fry basket in the oven.
11. When the cooking time is completed, remove the air fry basket from the oven and transfer the haddock steak onto a serving platter.
12. Immediately coat the haddock steaks with the remaining glaze.
13. Serve immediately alongside the spinach.

Nutritional Information per Serving:

Calories: 159
Fat: 1.4g
Carbohydrates: 4.7g
Fiber: 1g
Sugar: 2.3g
Protein: 31.5g
Sodium: 1100mg

Haddock with Tomatoes & Bell Peppers

Servings: 4
Preparation Time: 15 minutes
Cooking Time: 4 hours

Ingredients:

- 1 (15-ounce) can sugar-free diced tomatoes
- 1 green bell pepper, seeded and chopped
- 1 small onion, diced
- 1 garlic cloves, minced
- 1-pound haddock fillets
- 1 teaspoon dried herbs
- Salt and ground black pepper, as required
- 1/3 cup low-sodium chicken broth

Instructions:

1. Lightly grease a Dutch oven that will fit in the Breville Smart Air Fryer Oven.
2. In the greased pot, place the tomatoes, bell pepper, onion and garlic and stir to combine.
3. Place the fish fillets on top of the tomato mixture and sprinkle with the herbs, salt and black pepper.
4. Place the broth on top evenly.
5. Arrange the Dutch oven over the wire rack.
6. Select "Slow Cooker" of Breville Smart Air Fryer Oven and set on "High".
7. Set the timer for 4 hours and press "Start/Stop" to begin cooking.

8. When the cooking time is completed, remove the Dutch oven from the oven.

9. Remove the lid and serve hot.

Nutritional Information per Serving:

Calories: 165

Fat: 1.4g

Carbohydrates: 8.5g

Fiber: 2.2g

Sugar: 5.1g

Protein: 29.2g

Sodium: 150mg

Glazed Hake

Servings: 2
Preparation Time: 10 minutes
Cooking Time: 12 minutes

Ingredients:

- 4 tablespoons low-sodium soy sauce
- 2 tablespoons honey
- 3 teaspoons fresh lime juice
- I teaspoon water
- 4 (3½-ounce) hake fillets
- 2 cups fresh baby arugula
- I tomato, chopped

Instructions:

1. In a small bowl, mix together the soy sauce, honey, vinegar and water.
2. In another small bowl, reserve about half of the mixture.
3. Add the hake fillets in the remaining mixture and coat well.
4. Cover the bowl and refrigerate to marinate for about 2 hours.
5. Arrange the hake fillets into the greased air fry basket.
6. Select "Air Fry" of Breville Smart Air Fryer Oven and adjust the temperature to 355 degrees F.
7. Set the timer for 12 minutes and press "Start/Stop" to begin preheating.
8. When the unit beeps to show that it is preheated, insert the air fry basket in the oven.

9. Flip the hake fillets once halfway through and coat with the reserved marinade after every 3 minutes.

10. When the cooking time is completed, remove the hake fillets from the oven and transfer onto serving plates.

11. Serve hot alongside the arugula and tomato.

Nutritional Information per Serving:

Calories: 211
Fat: 1.6g
Carbohydrates: 20g
Fiber: 0.7g
Sugar: 20g
Protein: 30.9g
Sodium: 1289mg

Seasoned Catfish

Servings: 4
Preparation Time: 10 minutes
Cooking Time: 23 minutes

Ingredients:

- 4 (4-ounce) catfish fillets
- 2 tablespoons Italian seasoning
- Salt and ground black pepper, as required
- 1 tablespoon olive oil
- 6 cups fresh baby greens

Instructions:

1. Rub the fish fillets with seasoning, salt and black pepper generously and then, coat with oil.
2. Arrange the fish fillets into the greased air fry basket.
3. Select "Air Fry" of Breville Smart Air Fryer Oven and adjust the temperature to 400 degrees F.
4. Set the timer for 20 minutes and press "Start/Stop" to begin preheating.
5. When the unit beeps to show that it is preheated, insert the air fry basket in the oven.
6. Flip the fish fillets once halfway through.
7. When the cooking time is completed, remove the air fry basket from the oven and serve hot alongside the greens.

Nutritional Information per Serving:

Calories: 285
Fat: 13.9g
Carbohydrates: 4.9g
Fiber: 1.6g
Sugar: 2.1g
Protein: 32.2g
Sodium: 289mg

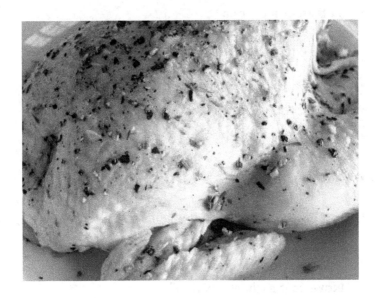

Cajun Catfish

Servings: 2
Preparation Time: 10 minutes
Cooking Time: 14 minutes

Ingredients:

- 2 tablespoons almond flour
- 2 teaspoons Cajun seasoning
- ½ teaspoon paprika
- ½ teaspoon garlic powder
- Salt, as required
- 2 (6-ounce) catfish fillets
- 1 tablespoon olive oil
- 3 cups fresh baby spinach

Instructions:

1. In a bowl, mix together the flour, Cajun seasoning, paprika, garlic powder, and salt.
2. Add the catfish fillets and coat with the mixture evenly.
3. Now, coat each fillet with oil.
4. Arrange the fish fillets into the greased air fry basket.
5. Select "Air Fry" of Breville Smart Air Fryer Oven and adjust the temperature to 400 degrees F.
6. Set the timer for 14 minutes and press "Start/Stop" to begin preheating.
7. When the unit beeps to show that it is preheated, insert the air fry basket in the oven.
8. Flip the fish fillets once halfway through.

9. When the cooking time is completed, remove the air fry basket from the oven and serve hot alongside the spinach.

Nutritional Information per Serving:

Calories: 349
Fat: 23.9g
Carbohydrates: 3.7g
Fiber: 2g
Sugar: 0.7g
Protein: 28g
Sodium: 254mg

Sardine in Tomato Gravy

Servings: 6
Preparation Time: 15 minutes
Cooking Time: 8 hours

Ingredients:

- 2 tablespoons olive oil
- 2 pounds fresh sardines, cubed
- 4 plum tomatoes, chopped finely
- 1 small onion, sliced
- 1 medium bell pepper, seeded and sliced
- 2 garlic cloves, minced
- 1 cup tomato puree
- Salt and ground black pepper, as required

Instructions:

1. In a baking dish, spread the oil evenly.
2. Place sardine over oil and top with the remaining all ingredients.
3. Arrange the baking dish over the wire rack.
4. Select "Slow Cooker" of Breville Smart Air Fryer Oven and set on "Low".
5. Set the timer for 8 hours and press "Start/Stop" to begin cooking.
6. When the cooking time is completed, remove the pan from the oven serve hot.

Nutritional Information per Serving:

Calories: 297
Fat: 16.7g
Carbohydrates: 7.2g
Fiber: 1.8g
Sugar: 3.9g
Protein: 29.2g
Sodium: 605mg

Tuna & Mustard Burgers

Servings: 4
Preparation Time: 15 minutes
Cooking Time: 6 minutes

Ingredients:

For Burgers:

- 7 ounces canned tuna
- 1 large egg
- ¼ cup breadcrumbs
- 1 tablespoon mustard
- ¼ teaspoon garlic powder
- ¼ teaspoon onion powder
- ¼ teaspoon cayenne pepper
- Salt and ground black pepper, as required

For Serving:

- 1 large cucumber, chopped
- 4 cups fresh baby spinach

Instructions:

1. For burgers: in a bowl, add all the ingredients and mix until well combined.
2. Make 4 equal-sized patties from the mixture.
3. Arrange the patties onto the greased enamel roasting pan.
4. Set the timer for 6 minutes and press "Start/Stop" to begin preheating.

5. When the unit beeps to show that it is preheated, insert the roasting pan in the oven.
6. Flip the burgers once halfway through.
7. When the cooking time is completed, remove the roasting pan from the oven and transfer the burgers onto serving plates.
8. Serve hot alongside the cucumber and spinach.

Nutritional Information per Serving:

Calories: 170
Fat: 6.6g
Carbohydrates: 10g
Fiber: 1.8g
Sugar: 2.2g
Protein: 17.7g
Sodium: 156mg

Tuna & Mayonnaise Burgers

Servings: 4
Preparation Time: 15 minutes
Cooking Time: 12 minutes

Ingredients:

- 2 (6-ounces) cans tuna, drained
- 1½ tablespoons low-fat mayonnaise
- 1½ tablespoon almond flour
- 1 tablespoon fresh lemon juice
- 1 teaspoon dried dill
- 1 teaspoon garlic powder
- ½ teaspoon onion powder
- Pinch of salt and ground black pepper
- 3 cups fresh salad greens
- 1 large tomato, chopped

Instructions:

1. In a large bowl, mix together the tuna, mayonnaise, flour, lemon juice, dill, and spices.
2. Make 4 equal-sized patties from the mixture.
3. Arrange the patties onto the greased enamel roasting pan.
4. Set the timer for 12 minutes and press "Start/Stop" to begin preheating.
5. When the unit beeps to show that it is preheated, insert the roasting pan in the oven.
6. Flip the burgers once halfway through.

7. When the cooking time is completed, remove the roasting pan from the oven and transfer the burgers onto serving plates.
8. Serve hot alongside the greens and tomatoes.

Nutritional Information per Serving:

Calories: 215
Fat: 10g
Carbohydrates: 5.8g
Fiber: 1.2g
Sugar: 2.4g
Protein: 23.4g
Sodium: 89mg

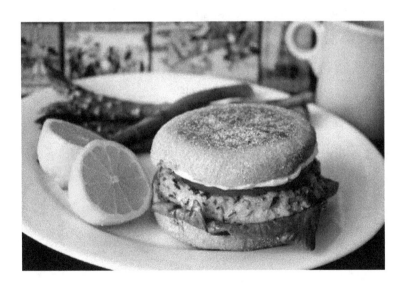

Prawn Burgers

Servings: 2
Preparation Time: 15 minutes
Cooking Time: 6 minutes

Ingredients:

For Burgers:

- ½ cup prawns, peeled, deveined and chopped very finely
- ½ cup breadcrumbs
- 2-3 tablespoons onion, chopped finely
- ½ teaspoon ginger, minced
- ½ teaspoon garlic, minced
- ½ teaspoon red chili powder
- ½ teaspoon ground cumin
- ¼ teaspoon ground turmeric
- Salt and ground black pepper, as required

For Serving:

- 2 cups fresh baby greens
- 1 cup cherry tomatoes, halved

Instructions:

1. For burgers: in a bowl, add all ingredients and mix until well combined.
2. Make small sized patties from mixture.
3. Arrange the patties into the greased air fry basket.

4. Select mode "Air Fry" on Air Fryer Oven and adjust the temperature to 355 degrees F.
5. Set the timer for 6 minutes and press "Start/Stop" to begin preheating.
6. When the unit beeps to show that it is preheated, insert the air fry basket in the oven.
7. When the cooking time is completed, remove the air fry basket from the oven and transfer the burgers onto serving plates.
8. Serve hot alongside the greens and tomatoes.

Nutritional Information per Serving:

Calories: 273
Fat: 3.8g
Carbohydrates: 255.1g
Fiber: 3.3g
Sugar: 4.9g
Protein: 31g
Sodium: 589mg

Prawns in Garlic Sauce

Servings: 2
Preparation Time: 15 minutes
Cooking Time: 6 minutes

Ingredients:

- ½ pound large prawns, peeled and deveined
- 1 large garlic clove, minced
- 1 tablespoon coconut oil, melted
- 1 teaspoon fresh lemon zest, grated
- 3 cups fresh baby kale

Instructions:

1. In a bowl, add all the ingredients except for baby kale and toss to coat well.
2. Set aside at room temperature for about 30 minutes.
3. Arrange the prawn mixture into a baking dish.
4. Select "Bake" of Breville Smart Air Fryer Oven and adjust the temperature to 450 degrees F.
5. Set the timer for 6 minutes and press "Start/Stop" to begin preheating.
6. When the unit beeps to show that it is preheated, arrange the baking dish over the wire rack.
7. When the cooking time is completed, remove the baking dish from the oven and transfer the shrimp onto serving plates.
8. Serve immediately alongside the baby kale.

Nutritional Information per Serving:

Calories: 240
Fat: 9.2g
Carbohydrates: 9g
Fiber: 1.6g
Sugar: 0.1g
Protein: 28.2g
Sodium: 303mg

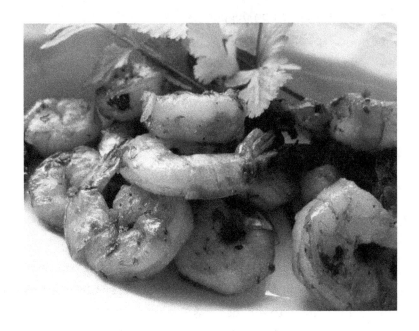

Lemony Shrimp

Servings: 3
Preparation Time: 15 minutes
Cooking Time: 8 minutes

Ingredients:

- 2 tablespoons fresh lemon juice
- 1 tablespoon olive oil
- 1 teaspoon lemon pepper
- ¼ teaspoon paprika
- ¼ teaspoon garlic powder
- 12 ounces medium shrimp, peeled and deveined
- 5 cups fresh spinach

Instructions:

1. In a large bowl, add all the ingredients except the shrimp and spinach mix until well combined.
2. Add the shrimp and toss to coat well.
3. Arrange the shrimps onto the enamel roasting pan.
4. Select "Air Fry" of Breville Smart Air Fryer Oven and adjust the temperature to 400 degrees F.
5. Set the timer for 8 minutes and press "Start/Stop" to begin preheating.
6. When the unit beeps to show that it is preheated, insert the roasting pan in the oven.
7. When the cooking time is completed, remove the roasting pan from the oven and transfer the shrimp onto serving plates.
8. Serve hot alongside the spinach.

Nutritional Information per Serving:

Calories: 192
Fat: 6.9g
Carbohydrates: 4.5g
Fiber: 1.4g
Sugar: 0.5g
Protein: 27.5g
Sodium: 319mg

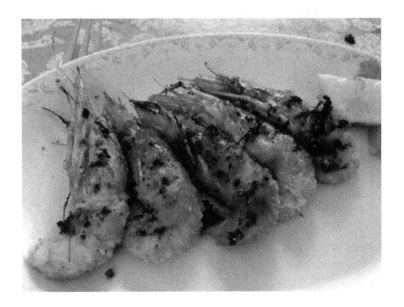

Parmesan Shrimp

Servings: 4
Preparation Time: 15 minutes
Cooking Time: 10 minutes

Ingredients:

- 2/3 cup low-fat Parmesan cheese, grated
- 4 garlic cloves, minced
- 2 tablespoons olive oil
- 1 teaspoon dried basil
- ½ teaspoon dried oregano
- 1 teaspoon onion powder
- ½ teaspoon red pepper flakes, crushed
- Ground black pepper, as required
- 2 pounds shrimp, peeled and deveined
- 1-2 tablespoons fresh lemon juice
- 6 cups fresh spinach

Instructions:

1. In a large bowl, add the Parmesan cheese, garlic, oil, herbs, and spices and mix well
2. Add the shrimp and toss to coat well.
3. Arrange the shrimp into the greased air fry basket.
4. Select "Air Fry" of Breville Smart Air Fryer Oven and adjust the temperature to 350 degrees F.
5. Set the timer for 10 minutes and press "Start/Stop" to begin preheating.

6. When the unit beeps to show that it is preheated, insert the air fry basket in the oven.
7. When the cooking time is completed, remove the air fry basket from the oven and transfer the shrimp onto a platter.
8. Drizzle with lemon juice and serve immediately alongside the spinach.

Nutritional Information per Serving:

Calories: 262
Fat: 9.6g
Carbohydrates: 4.7g
Fiber: 0.8g
Sugar: 0.4g
Protein: 37.7g
Sodium: 564mg

Shrimp with Tomatoes

Servings: 4
Preparation Time: 15 minutes
Cooking Time: 7¼ hours

Ingredients:

- 1 (14-ounce) can peeled tomatoes, chopped finely
- 4 ounces canned tomato paste
- 2 garlic cloves, minced
- 2 tablespoons fresh parsley, chopped
- Salt and ground black pepper, as required
- 1 teaspoon lemon pepper
- 2 pounds cooked shrimp, peeled and deveined

Instructions:

1. In an oven-safe pan that will fit in the Breville Smart Air Fryer Oven, place all ingredients except for shrimp and stir to combine.
2. Cover the pan with a lid.
3. Arrange the pan over the wire rack.
4. Select "Slow Cooker" of Breville Smart Air Fryer Oven and set on "Low".
5. Set the timer for 7 hours and press "Start/Stop" to begin cooking.
6. When the cooking time is completed, remove the pan from the oven.
7. Remove the lid and stir in the shrimp.
8. Again, arrange the pan over the wire rack.

9. Select "Slow Cooker" of Breville Smart Air Fryer Oven and set on "High".
10. Set the timer for 15 minutes and press "Start/Stop" to begin cooking.
11. When the cooking time is completed, remove the pan from the oven.
12. Remove the lid and stir and serve hot.

Nutritional Information per Serving:

Calories: 315
Fat: 4.2g
Carbohydrates: 12.6g
Fiber: 2.6g
Sugar: 6g
Protein: 54g
Sodium: 625mg

Shrimp Kabobs

Servings: 2
Preparation Time: 15 minutes
Cooking Time: 8 minutes

Ingredients:

- ¾ pound shrimp, peeled and deveined
- 2 tablespoons fresh lemon juice
- 1 teaspoon garlic, minced
- ½ teaspoon paprika
- ½ teaspoon ground cumin
- Salt and ground black pepper, as required
- 1 tablespoon fresh cilantro, chopped
- 3 cups fresh arugula

Instructions:

1. In a bowl, mix together the lemon juice, garlic, and spices.
2. Add the shrimp and mix well.
3. Thread the shrimp onto presoaked wooden skewers.
4. Arrange the skewers into the greased air fry basket.
5. Select "Air Fry" of Breville Smart Air Fryer Oven and adjust the temperature to 350 degrees F.
6. Set the timer for 8 minutes and press "Start/Stop" to begin preheating.
7. When the unit beeps to show that it is preheated, insert the air fry basket in the oven.
8. Flip the skewers once halfway through.

9. When the cooking time is completed, remove the air fry basket from the oven and transfer the shrimp kebabs onto serving plates.

10. Garnish with fresh cilantro and serve immediately alongside the arugula.

Calories: 219
Fat: 3.4g
Carbohydrates: 5g
Fiber: 0.8g
Sugar: 1g
Protein: 39.9g
Sodium: 505mg

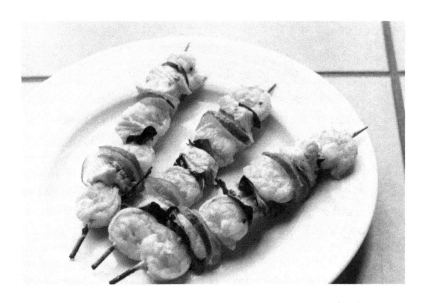

Herbed Scallops

Servings: 2
Preparation Time: 15 minutes
Cooking Time: 4 minutes

Ingredients:

- ¾ pound sea scallops, cleaned and pat dry
- 1 tablespoon coconut oil, melted
- ¼ tablespoon fresh thyme, minced
- ¼ tablespoon fresh rosemary, minced
- Salt and ground black pepper, as required
- 3 cups fresh arugula

Instructions:

1. In a large bowl, place the scallops, coconut oil, herbs, salt, and black pepper and toss to coat well.
2. Arrange the scallops into the greased air fry basket.
3. Select "Air Fry" of Breville Smart Air Fryer Oven and adjust the temperature to 390 degrees F.
4. Set the timer for 4 minutes and press "Start/Stop" to begin preheating.
5. When the unit beeps to show that it is preheated, insert the air fry basket in the oven.
6. When the cooking time is completed, remove the air fry basket from the oven.
7. Serve hot alongside the arugula.

Nutritional Information per Serving:

Calories: 218
Fat: 8.4g
Carbohydrates: 5.6g
Fiber: 0.8g
Sugar: 0.6g
Protein: 29.4g
Sodium: 360mg

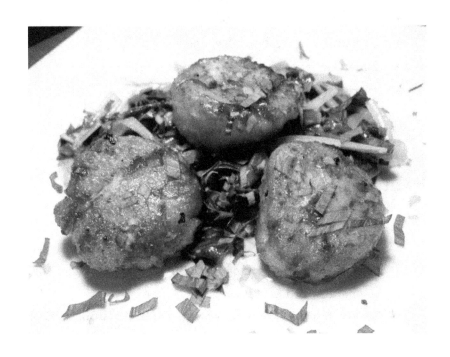

Scallops with Capers Sauce

Servings: 2
Preparation Time: 15 minutes
Cooking Time: 6 minutes

Ingredients:

- 10 (1-ounce) sea scallops, cleaned and patted very dry
- Salt and ground black pepper, as required
- ¼ cup extra-virgin olive oil
- 2 tablespoons fresh parsley, finely chopped
- 2 teaspoons capers, finely chopped
- 1 teaspoon fresh lemon zest, finely grated
- ½ teaspoon garlic, finely chopped
- 3 cups fresh baby spinach

Instructions:

1. Season each scallop evenly with salt and black pepper.
2. Arrange scallops into the greased air fry basket in a single layer.
3. Select "Air Fry" of Breville Smart Air Fryer Oven and adjust the temperature to 400 degrees F.
4. Set the timer for 6 minutes and press "Start/Stop" to begin preheating.
5. When the unit beeps to show that it is preheated, insert the air fry basket in the oven.
6. Meanwhile, for the sauce: in a bowl, add the remaining ingredients except for spinach and mix well.
7. When the cooking time is completed, remove the air fry basket from the oven and transfer the scallops onto serving plates.

8. Top with the sauce and serve immediately alongside the spinach.

Nutritional Information per Serving:

Calories: 237
Fat: 17.7g
Carbohydrates: 3.9g
Fiber: 0.9g
Sugar: 0.2g
Protein: 16.9g
Sodium: 284mg

Scallops with Spinach

Servings: 3
Preparation Time: 15 minutes
Cooking Time: 10 minutes

Ingredients:

- 1 (12-ounces) package frozen spinach, thawed and drained
- 12 jumbo sea scallops
- Olive oil cooking spray
- Salt and ground black pepper, as required
- ¾ cup low-fat cream
- 1 tablespoon tomato paste
- 1 teaspoon garlic, minced
- 1 tablespoon fresh basil, chopped

Instructions:

1. In the bottom of a 7-inch heatproof pan, place the spinach.
2. Spray each scallop evenly with cooking spray and then, sprinkle with a little salt and black pepper.
3. Arrange scallops on top of the spinach in a single layer.
4. In a bowl, add the cream, tomato paste, garlic, basil, salt, and black pepper and mix well.
5. Place the cream mixture over the spinach and scallops evenly.
6. Arrange the pan into the air fry basket.
7. Select "Air Fry" of Breville Smart Air Fryer Oven and adjust the temperature to 350 degrees F.
8. Set the timer for 10 minutes and press "Start/Stop" to begin preheating.

9. When the unit beeps to show that it is preheated, insert the air fry basket in the oven.

10. When the cooking time is completed, remove the air fry basket from the oven and serve hot.

Nutritional Information per Serving:

Calories: 257
Fat: 6.1g
Carbohydrates: 15g
Fiber: 4.1g
Sugar: 1.8g
Protein: 36.9g
Sodium: 536mg

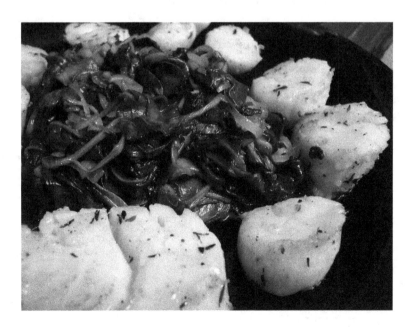

Crab Cakes

Servings: 4
Preparation Time: 15 minutes
Cooking Time: 10 minutes

Ingredients:

- 1-pound lump crab meat
- 1/3 cup panko breadcrumbs
- ¼ cup scallion, finely chopped
- 2 large eggs
- 2 tablespoons low-fat mayonnaise
- 1 teaspoon Dijon mustard
- 1 teaspoon Worcestershire sauce
- 1½ teaspoons Old Bay seasoning
- Ground black pepper, as required
- 6 cups fresh baby greens

Instructions:

1. In a large bowl, add all the ingredients and gently stir to combine.
2. Cover the bowl and refrigerate for about 1 hour.
3. Make 8 equal-sized patties from the mixture.
4. Arrange the crab cakes into the greased air fry basket.
5. Select "Air Fry" of Breville Smart Air Fryer Oven and adjust the temperature to 375 degrees F.
6. Set the timer for 10 minutes and press "Start/Stop" to begin preheating.
7. When the unit beeps to show that it is preheated, insert the air fry basket in the oven.

8. Flip the crab cakes once halfway through.

9. When the cooking time is completed, remove the air fry basket from the oven and serve alongside the greens.

Nutritional Information per Serving:

Calories: 176
Fat: 14.4g
Carbohydrates: 9.3g
Fiber: 1.4g
Sugar: 1.3g
Protein: 21g
Sodium: 889mg

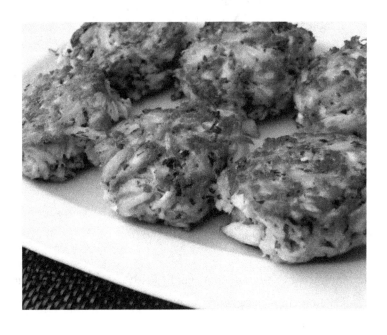

Herbed Seafood Stew

Servings: 8
Preparation Time: 20 minutes
Cooking Time: 4¾ hours

Ingredients:

- 1 small celery stalk, chopped
- 1 small carrot, peeled and chopped
- 1 yellow onion, chopped
- 3 garlic cloves, chopped
- 1 cup fresh cilantro leaves, chopped
- 1 cup tomatoes, chopped finely
- 4 cups chicken broth
- 2 tablespoons fresh lemon juice
- 2 tablespoons olive oil
- 3 teaspoons mixed dried herbs (rosemary, thyme, marjoram)
- Salt and ground black pepper, as required
- 1-pound cod fillets, cubed
- 1-pound shrimp, peeled and deveined
- 1-pound scallops
- ¾ cup crabmeat

Instructions:

1. In an oven-safe pan that will fit in the Breville Smart Air Fryer Oven, place all ingredients except for seafood and stir to combine.
2. Cover the pan with a lid.
3. Arrange the pan over the wire rack.

4. Select "Slow Cooker" of Breville Smart Air Fryer Oven and set on "Low".
5. Set the timer for 4 hours and press "Start/Stop" to begin cooking.
6. When the cooking time is completed, remove the pan from the oven.
7. Open the lid and stir in the seafood.
8. Cover the pan with a lid.
9. Arrange the pan over the wire rack.
10. Select "Slow Cooker" of Breville Smart Air Fryer Oven and set on "Low".
11. Set the timer for 45 minutes and press "Start/Stop" to begin cooking.
12. When the cooking time is completed, remove the pan from the oven and stir the mixture well.
13. Serve hot.

Nutritional Information per Serving:

Calories: 228
Fat: 6.3g
Carbohydrates: 5.6g
Fiber: 0.8g
Sugar: 1.7g
Protein: 35.8g
Sodium: 687mg

Seafood & Tomato Stew

Servings: 8
Preparation Time: 20 minutes
Cooking Time: 4 hours 50 minutes

Ingredients:

- 2 tablespoons olive oil
- 1-pound tomatoes, chopped
- 1 large yellow onion, chopped finely
- 2 garlic cloves, minced
- 2 teaspoons curry powder
- 6 sprigs fresh parsley
- Salt and ground black pepper, as required
- 1½ cups low-sodium chicken broth
- 1½ pounds salmon, cut into cubes
- 1½ pounds shrimp, peeled and deveined

Instructions:

1. In an oven-safe pan that will fit in the Breville Smart Air Fryer Oven, place all ingredients except for seafood and stir to combine.
2. Cover the pan with a lid.
3. Arrange the pan over the wire rack.
4. Select "Slow Cooker" of Breville Smart Air Fryer Oven and set on "High".
5. Set the timer for 4 hours and press "Start/Stop" to begin cooking.

6. When the cooking time is completed, remove the pan from the oven.
7. Remove the lid and stir in the seafood.
8. Cover the pan with a lid.
9. Again, arrange the pan over the wire rack.
10. Select "Slow Cooker" of Breville Smart Air Fryer Oven and set on "Low".
11. Set the timer for 50 minutes and press "Start/Stop" to begin cooking.
12. When the cooking time is completed, remove the pan from the oven.
13. Remove the lid and stir the mixture well.
14. Serve hot.

Nutritional Information per Serving:

Calories: 267
Fat: 10.4g
Carbohydrates: 6g
Fiber: 1.3g
Sugar: 2.3g
Protein: 37.1g
Sodium: 282mg

Seafood & Spinach Stew

Servings: 8
Preparation Time: 20 minutes
Cooking Time: 4 hours 50 minutes

Ingredients:

- 2 tablespoons olive oil
- ½ pound tomatoes, chopped
- 1 large yellow onion, chopped finely
- 2 garlic cloves, minced
- 2 teaspoons curry powder
- 6 sprigs fresh parsley
- Salt and ground black pepper, as required
- 1½ cups chicken broth
- 1½ pounds salmon, cut into cubes
- 1½ pounds shrimp, peeled and deveined
- 1-pound fresh spinach, chopped

Instructions:

1. In an oven-safe pan that will fit in the Breville Smart Air Fryer Oven, place all ingredients except for seafood and spinach and stir to combine.
2. Cover the pan with a lid.
3. Arrange the pan over the wire rack.
4. Select "Slow Cooker" of Breville Smart Air Fryer Oven and set on "Low".
5. Set the timer for 4 hours and press "Start/Stop" to begin cooking.

6. When the cooking time is completed, remove the pan from the oven.
7. Open the lid and stir in the seafood and spinach.
8. Cover the pan with a lid.
9. Arrange the pan over the wire rack.
10. Select "Slow Cooker" of Breville Smart Air Fryer Oven and set on "Low".
11. Set the timer for 50 minutes and press "Start/Stop" to begin cooking.
12. When the cooking time is completed, remove the pan from the oven and serve hot.

Calories: 279
Fat: 10.8g
Carbohydrates: 6.9g
Fiber: 2.2g
Sugar: 1.9g
Protein: 39g
Sodium: 455mg

Seafood with Zucchini Noodles

Servings: 4
Preparation Time: 15 minutes
Cooking Time: 8 minutes

Ingredients:

- 4 tablespoons pesto, divided
- 4 (4-ounce) salmon steaks
- 2 tablespoons olive oil
- ½ pound cherry tomatoes, chopped
- 8 large prawns, peeled and deveined
- 2 tablespoons fresh lemon juice
- 2 tablespoons fresh thyme, chopped
- 2 large zucchinis, spiralized with Blade C

Instructions:

1. In the bottom of a baking pan, spread 1 tablespoon of pesto.
2. Place the salmon steaks and tomatoes over pesto in a single layer and drizzle evenly with the oil.
3. Now, place the prawns on top in a single layer.
4. Drizzle with lemon juice and sprinkle with thyme.
5. Arrange the pan into the air fry basket.
6. Select "Air Fry" of Breville Smart Air Fryer Oven and adjust the temperature to 390 degrees F.
7. Set the timer for 8 minutes and press "Start/Stop" to begin preheating.
8. When the unit beeps to show that it is preheated, insert the air fry basket in the oven.

9. When the cooking time is completed, remove the air fry basket from the oven and transfer the salmon mixture into a bowl.
10. Add the remaining pesto and toss to coat well.
11. Divide the zucchini noodles onto serving plates and top with salmon mixture.
12. Serve immediately.

Nutritional Information per Serving:

Calories: 371
Fat: 21.8g
Carbohydrates: 10g
Fiber: 3.2g
Sugar: 5g
Protein: 36.2g
Sodium: 274mg

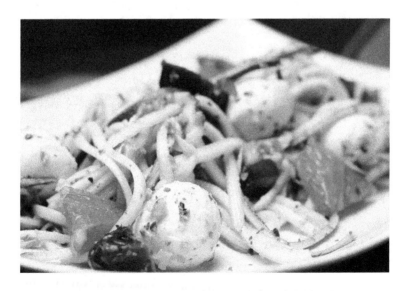

CPSIA information can be obtained
at www.ICGtesting.com
Printed in the USA
BVHW090851140621
609525BV00002B/69

9 781803 218113